KETOGENIC DIET FOR BEGINNERS:

Lose a Lot of Weight Fast Using Your Body's Natural Processes

Charlie Mason

Table of Contents

The following eBook is reproduced below with the goal of providing information that is as accurate and reliable as possible. Regardless, purchasing this eBook can be seen as consent to the fact that both the publisher and the author of this book are in no way experts on the topics discussed within and that any recommendations or suggestions that are made herein are for entertainment purposes only. Professionals should be consulted as needed prior to undertaking any of the action endorsed herein.

This declaration is deemed fair and valid by both the American Bar Association and the Committee of Publishers Association and is legally binding throughout the United States.

Furthermore, the transmission, duplication or reproduction of any of the following work including specific information will be considered an illegal act irrespective of if it is done electronically or in print. This extends to creating a secondary or tertiary copy of the work or a recorded copy and is only allowed with express written consent of the Publisher. All additional right reserved.

The information in the following pages is broadly considered to be a truthful and accurate account of facts and as such any inattention, use or misuse of the information in question by the reader will render any resulting actions solely under their purview. There are no scenarios in which the publisher or the original author of this work can be in any fashion deemed liable for any hardship or damages that may befall them after undertaking information described herein.

Additionally, the information in the following pages is intended only for informational purposes and should thus be thought of as universal. As befitting its nature, it is presented without assurance regarding its prolonged validity or interim quality. Trademarks that are mentioned are done without written consent and can in no way be considered an endorsement from the trademark holder.

Introduction

Congratulations on getting this book and thank you for doing so.

The following chapters will discuss how to use the ketogenic diet to achieve your weight loss goals.

There are plenty of books on this subject on the market, thanks again for choosing this one! Every effort was made to ensure it is full of as much useful information as possible, please enjoy!

CHAPTER 1

How Ketosis Can Benefit You

If I told you that your body had a natural system for burning fat that you simply weren't utilizing, would you believe me? Most people wouldn't. However, more and more people are coming around to this wonderful diet in what I like to call the low-carb revolution.

The purpose of the ketogenic diet is to retrain your body to run on better fuel. Rather than glucose, your body will learn to run on fat for fuel. Eating this way will place your body in a position wherein it primarily uses fat, rather than sugar for energy.

However, the ketogenic diet is focused on one key concept: *ketosis*. *Ketosis* is, to simply say, an alternative way that the body can burn fuel. When one is in a state of *ketosis*, then they are burning what are called *ketones* for energy, instead of *carbohydrates* like usual. Ketones can be generated from both the body's fat deposits and stores, as well as from ingested fat. This leads us to the first way that ketosis can benefit you: you'll be *less hungry*. We'll talk more about the simple mechanics of weight loss either, but for right now, just understand this: fats burn *slower* than carbs do, which means that you'll be a lot less hungry a lot less often.

Moreover, when you're eating *less* energy than your body is taking out, your body takes energy *directly* from your natural fat stores without any sort of conversion process, meaning that you'll shed pounds like crazy.

When you eat a diet that is heavy in carbohydrates-grains, sugars, starches, vegetables, fruits- you are feeding your body a ton of glucose. Your body stores this glucose away as glycogen in the liver and muscles for later use. The glucose stored in the liver can be used by most systems in the body. The glucose stored in your muscles can only be used by the specific muscle it is stored in. However, your body can store only a limited amount of glucose.

Ketosis can also help with your blood pressure. Ketosis, in a word, causes you to pee – a *lot.* This means that your body requires a lot more water. However, in this heavier urination, you also shed a lot more electrolytes, meaning that your sodium levels can go down massively which will benefit your blood pressure.

The simple idea behind ketosis and the ketogenic diet is simply taking in fat as your main source of cholesterol. One may think that this seems counterintuitive to helping one's blood pressure and general health. However, it's quite the opposite. If you were to run lab tests after having a healthy ketogenic diet for six months, you would find that your lipid levels were higher, your bad cholesterol levels were lower, your good cholesterol levels were higher, and your blood pressure is lower and far more stable than it may have been before. In other words, your blood becomes a lot healthier – and so do you!

CHAPTER 2

What to Expect on Keto

So now that we've talked about what ketosis is, what can you expect on a ketogenic diet? Well, this is actually pretty simple to breakdown.

Firstly, you should expect *rapid weight loss*. People often turn to low-carb diets such as keto because they see the success that others have had with their personal low-carb adventures, and they decide that they'd like to see similar results. This is completely understandable; clinical tests comparing low-carb and low-fat diets have found that people following a low-carb diet will show greater amounts of weight loss at 6 months than those following a low-fat diet.

You will also lose a fair bit of water weight in the first week while your body uses up its glycogen reserves for energy (essentially, what was left over from your body's carbohydrate stores). It's not uncommon for somebody to lose 7 to 10 pounds in their first week in water weight. After this initial period, you should see a steady loss of 1 to 2 pounds per week, potentially more depending upon factors such as age and how your body personally processes energy.

This leads us to the next thing that we have to talk about: *keto flu*. This is an unfortunate affliction that most people starting keto have to deal with. What is essentially happening is a combination of electrolyte imbalance alongside dehydration.

It's simple enough, but can make you feel just like you have the flu!

Ketosis, as I said, is diuretic. You're going to have to account for this by drinking a whole lot of water. You're also going to be peeing out a lot of your body's electrolytes, or losing them through other channels in greater amounts. This means that you need to replace them. You'll want to salt your food quite heavily, and also take potassium and magnesium supplements.

If the keto flu gets particularly bad, many find that drinking chicken broth can help them overcome the symptoms of keto flu for a while. This is because chicken broth is rather high in sodium and, of course, is water-based. The combination of these can restore a bit of your body's natural order. In other words, chicken broth can help you to feel better for much the same reason that it did when you drank it as a child to help with the common cold!

One of the reasons that people particularly like low-carb diets for weight loss is because they leave you feeling a lot less hungry. Carbs and fats are burned differently by the body. Fats take longer to process and go further, while carbs tend to be burned very quickly and used in one go. This is why carbs can leave you feeling tired or you get a "sugar high". Fats don't come with that; rather, they leave you feeling full for longer. This means that while other diets might leave you feeling hungry and tired, the ketogenic diet will leave you feeling more energetic and will hardly leave you hungry. It wouldn't be uncommon if you didn't feel like eating breakfast simply because you weren't hungry.

CHAPTER 3

Principles of Weight Loss

I've tried to help a lot of people lose weight, and I've discussed weight loss likewise with a lot of people. I've heard a lot of people make a *lot* of excuses. People could say that, for example, no matter what they do, they just *can't* lose weight for some reason. It's always the same set of excuses - "I simply can't lose weight"; "my body isn't wired for it"; "my metabolism is too slow"; it's the same set of tired diatribes that have little basis in reality.

However, the truth is, weight loss comes down to a simple equation of calories in versus calories out. Although there are certain other factors which may play a part, such as your age or any medications you're on, weight loss, in general, comes down to a simple argument of burned energy. If you eat more calories than you burn, you'll gain weight; if you eat fewer calories than you burn, you'll lose weight.

Your body has a certain amount of calories that it burns as a result of your natural biological processes. This is referred to as your **basal metabolic rate**. This will vary depending on things such as your height, weight, and age. However, these are the calories which you burn without any effort on your end at all!

A lot of people think that you have to be an active person in order to lose weight. This isn't actually the truth. In order to lose weight, you simply have to eat fewer calories than you burn. As long as you eat less than your metabolic rate, you will lose weight. However, it's worth adding that working out is a major boon to your process of getting healthier. Losing weight is only one aspect of a much bigger spider web of increasing your overall physical health. Working out allows you to maintain your muscle mass that you've already got so that your body doesn't burn it off, and also allows you to tone up as you go.

CHAPTER 4

Starting Keto, Step by Step

So now we've talked about the various benefits of starting keto. The question then arises of how to start with keto - and, perhaps more importantly, where to start.

There are two different methods by which you can start keto: you can either start abruptly, or you can ease yourself into it. Many people find that doing the latter is the best means of beating keto flu.

The key thing to remember about starting any diet is that a successful diet isn't a simple dietary change; a successful diet is a holistic lifestyle change. In order to lose weight successfully, you're going to need to change the way you think about food entirely and simply consider it as fuel rather than a leisure activity.

However, combining this alongside a calorie deficit (which most people aren't used to eating at) and an entirely new way of eating can prove to be too much of a shock for many people. This can turn them off of the diet.

If you're not in too much of a rush to lose weight for a wedding or vacation, then consider easing into keto one thing at a time so that you aren't shocking yourself too much.

There are two different forms of keto, known as *strict keto and lazy keto* respectively.

Strict keto is a tightly controlled form of keto which allows you to eat within tightly controlled *macros*. Macros is short for macronutrients - fat, protein, and carbohydrates. The typical diet contains somewhere along the lines of ten percent fat, thirty percent protein, and sixty percent carbohydrates. On strict keto, however, you'd be eating sixty-five percent fat, twenty percent protein, and ten percent carbohydrates.

Lazy keto is simply the maintenance of ketosis by eating less than twenty grams of carbs per day. You can eat at a deficit or not; lazy keto is simply intended for maintenance of the diet and of ketosis.

Which one you decide to do is up to you. Some people work better and are able to stay more on track when they're taking advantage of a tighter regime, such as strict keto. On the other hand, some people find the freedom that lazy keto allows to be better for them personally. Whichever you prefer is the one you should use.

This chapter is specifically dedicated to easing into the ketogenic diet and setting yourself up for success using strict keto.

The first thing that you're going to want to do is figure out what deficit you're wanting to eat at. This can be done quite easily by simply calculating your basal metabolic rate. For calculating your basal metabolic rate, all that you will need are your age, weight, and height. I'm not going to make you do the math, but unfortunately, Amazon isn't kind to links in eBooks - Google "calculate BMR" and you'll be set.

Your basal metabolic rate, as we established in the last chapter, is the number of calories that you burn by simply existing. These are effortless calories. You can lead a sedentary lifestyle and as long as you're eating fewer than this number of calories per day, you *will* lose weight.

At this point, you can also set up a MyFitnessPal account. MyFitnessPal will automatically calculate your basal metabolic rate based on the information you provide. It will also automatically adjust how many calories you should have per day by how many pounds per week you say you'd like to lose. MyFitnessPal lets you log your meals and keep track of how many calories you eat, and you *will* need one if you decide to do strict keto. It's super easy to take anywhere because there's an easy-to-use mobile app for MyFitnessPal on both iOS and Android.

If you opt not to create a MyFitnessPal account and get the application, you're going to need to instead calculate how much of a deficit you need to eat at. I'd recommend only aiming to lose two pounds per week at most. A deficit beyond this is dangerous. There are 3500 calories in one pound, so in order to lose one pound, you must eat at a weekly deficit of 3500 calories or roughly a deficit of 500 calories per day. This means that if your basal metabolic rate is 2200 calories, you'll need to eat only 1700 to 1800 per day in order to lose a pound per week. One and a half pounds per week is a deficit of 750 calories, and two pounds per week is a deficit of 1000 calories. After you account for a 1000 calorie deficit, you're getting into starvation range, which is dangerous.

For the record, should you choose not to follow the steps outlined afterward, you can enter into ketosis by eating below fifty grams of carbs per day. However, the most rapid way is to eat below twenty grams of carbs per day, plus eating sub-twenty allows you to be 100% certain that you're going into ketosis.

Anyhow, moving forward. After figuring out your calorie deficit and learning how to account for the weight that you need to lose, as well as potentially setting up a MyFitnessPal account, you'll be ready to move to the next lesson. The next lesson involves how to read labels specifically for keto. Learning to read calories is not only important but absolutely vital, sure, and you'll want to pay attention to how many calories you consume. However, the best way to ease into keto is by simply becoming *aware* of carbs. Start reading labels of foods that you eat to look for their carbohydrates. This will also get you used to the idea of *net carbs*, which is central to keto. Net carbs are comprised of the carbs you eat which affect blood glucose. This means that the carbohydrates which don't affect blood glucose are unimportant. These may be listed as dietary fiber, sugar alcohols, or any other number of things. If you aren't sure, run a Google search to learn whether or not the term affects blood glucose. To draw the net carbs, you just deduct the grams of dietary fiber and sugar alcohols from the total carbohydrates. The goal on Keto is to eat fewer than twenty grams of net carbs per day; other forms of carbohydrate don't matter, as they don't affect blood sugar, they are simply passed.

The first step to actually transitioning to keto should be to eliminate your sweet tongue. I've found a lot of people from other cultures find it bizarre how many sweets we eat; indeed, once you wean yourself off of sugar, foods that you ate before start to seem *too* sweet by comparison.

You can do this first by eliminating any sodas. Replace them with diet sodas or sparkling water. This is a massive step for a lot of people. Our entire food culture is hugely reliant upon sodas to the point that we have a national coke addiction. Cut it out, and you'll notice a lot of different benefits.

After cutting out sodas, it's time to start cutting down on your snacking habits. Pay attention to them, first and foremost. If you notice that you feel like you're always snacking and subconsciously eating chips all the time, you drastically need to cut down on that. One of the biggest reasons for weight gain is constant snacking and boredom eating.

Again, weight loss has to do with mentality and how you think about food. Most people who are skinny aren't skinny because of their metabolism. Most people who are skinny are so because they don't derive as much pleasure from food, and see it more as fuel. You need to start thinking about food as fuel if you want to see a reasonable change in your weight.

There's no reason to boredom eat, whatsoever. Eating should be a conscious and mindful activity. Think about what you're eating, when you are. Eat slowly and consider the taste and feeling. You will feel fuller.

I'm sorry, but there's no compromise on this one. You either quit constantly snacking, or you aren't going to lose weight. It's a bad habit and one that should be broken. It's one thing if instead of three meals per day, you snack throughout the day, but if that's not the case then you need to cut out snacks. Calories add up too quickly. The only case in which you can make an exception is if you lead an active lifestyle.

After cutting out snacking, you're even closer to losing weight using keto. The next thing you're going to want to cut out is all dairy aside from heavy cream, half and half, and cheese without sugar added. This means that if you're a big milk drinker, you're going to be cutting it out at this point - sorry! It also means that if you eat cereal for breakfast on a daily basis you're going to need to find an alternative, such as eggs and bacon.

Next, you're going to want to cut out bread and other grains. This means you'll be saying goodbye to bread, rice, oatmeal, and any related foods. This can be a hard step, just consider breaking your portions in half at first. Order burgers with one bun instead of two, for example.

After cutting out bread and grains, you're most of the way there. The last big thing to cut out is fruit. While there are some fruits, like blueberries, which have a relatively low carb count, it may be easier to cut them out entirely. They serve as too much of a temptation and it becomes very difficult to constantly measure out exact servings.

At this point, you've dwindled it down to meat, cheese, vegetables, and nuts. Good. You're now, mostly, eating keto. One more thing you'll want to be wary of is that you should primarily be eating leafy vegetables and greens. Beware of lentils and beans as they have a huge number of carbs. Additionally, this is when you need to start cutting starches out of your diet almost entirely. Starches are things like potatoes. You do not need them, and they only serve to give you unnecessary carbs. Don't worry though; almost every starch has a nice keto replacement.

Transitioning to keto can be rather difficult; this isn't supposed to be a process that you undertake all at once. It can be nauseating if you try to do so. Rather, take a week on each step so you slowly adjust. Again, this is a *lifestyle* change, not just a diet.

CHAPTER 5

Sample Keto Recipes

Here are sample recipes you can use when you're starting off with keto.

Southwest Bacon Omelet

You'll need:

- 3 eggs
- 4 strips bacon
- ½ small onion
- 1 jalapeño
- ¼ cup cheddar cheese, shredded

1. Grill bacon in a skillet until cooked. Remove from the skillet and let it cool.

2. Chop jalapeño and onion, then sauté in bacon grease. Remove from the heat and place with the bacon.

3. Add olive oil to the pan in order to coat, then drain off the fat combination.

4. Crack and scramble eggs then place in a pan. Allow to cook for a moment, then add all ingredients.

5. Fold over omelet and let it cook for 1 minute on either side.

6. Serve and enjoy!

Calories: 630

Fat: 60g

Protein: 22g

Carbs: 4g

Zucchini Circles with Olive Garlic Sauce

You'll need:

- 2 zucchinis
- 2 oz smoked cheddar cheese
- ½ large onion
- 1 clove garlic
- 1 jalapeño
- Fresh cilantro
- ½ tomato
- Olive oil

1. Cut zucchini into thin circles. Roast 1 zucchini in the oven at 350 degrees for 30 minutes, flipping halfway. Set other to the side.
2. Meanwhile, prepare onion, garlic, and jalapeño by chopping.
3. Grill onion, garlic, and jalapeño in olive oil.
4. Add in roasted zucchini and grill together.

5. Add salt and pepper liberally.

6. Add smoked cheddar cheese and olive oil. Let cheddar melt. Squeeze tomato to get juices out. Set aside and chop remaining flesh.

7. Remove from the heat. Add cilantro, remaining zucchini, and tomato. Stir.

Calories: 470

Fat: 45g

Protein: 15g

Carbs: 6g

Crispy Flaxseed Waffles

You'll need:

- 2 cups ground flaxseed
- 1 tablespoon baking powder
- 1 teaspoon sea salt
- 5 tablespoons finely ground flaxseed with 15 tablespoons of warm water. Let it sit for 5 minutes until it's gooey (to replace eggs).
- ½ cup water
- ⅓ cup avocado oil or extra-virgin olive oil or melted coconut oil
- 2 teaspoons ground cinnamon

1. Heat waffle maker to medium high

2. In a large bowl, combine flax seed with baking powder and sea salt. Whisk to combine fully and set aside.

3. Add egg substitute, water and oil to a blender and blend on high for 30 seconds, until foamy.

4. Transfer liquid mixture to the bowl with the flaxseed mixture.

5. Stir to incorporate. The mixture will be very fluffy. Once incorporated, allow to sit for 3 minutes.

6. Toss in ground cinnamon.

7. Divide mixture into 4 servings. Scoop each; one at a time, onto the preheated waffle maker and close the top. Cook till done and repeat with remaining batter.

8. Serve warm or freeze in an air-tight container for a couple of weeks.

Calories: 297

Fat: 16g

Protein: 8.9g

Carbs: 8.4g

Those are just sample recipes to help get you started. Get creative in the kitchen!

CHAPTER 6

Sample Keto Shopping List

There are a lot of different keto recipes out there, so it's very difficult to pin down a shopping list or an exact set of items that you'll need. However, there are a few sample guidelines you should absolutely follow.

The first is that you're going to want primarily products which, obviously, are low carb and high fat. This will include meats, cheeses, and nuts. However, you're also going to want to grab a lot of leafy greens and vegetables that you can cook up and prepare.

Here is a sample list that you can use when doing ketogenic shopping:

- Lunch meat
- Ground beef
- Bacon
- Raw chicken, pork
- Cheddar cheese
- Mozzarella cheese
- Cream cheese
- Colby jack cheese
- Butter (grass-fed preferably)
- Olive oil
- Heavy cream -Half and half
- Coffee or tea
- Lots of water
- Spinach
- Broccoli

- Cauliflower

- Jalapeño pepper

- Yellow onion (use sparingly)

- Tomato (use sparingly)

- Garlic

- Eggs

Of course, you may also find recipes online that you'd like to try making. These will add items to your necessary grocery shopping. These are just basic requirements that will push you happy and healthy through your first week or two of keto.

CHAPTER 7

What to Eat and What Not to Eat

One of the hardest things about keto can be learning what you can and cannot eat. Indeed, this can be a little bit difficult. However, it's not totally horrible. It just takes a little bit of effort!

First, as should be perfectly clear, you aren't going to be eating any fruits or sugars. If something contains either, you aren't going to eat it. The same goes for starches. Don't eat any potatoes, sweet potatoes, or plant roots in general. These are loaded with carbs and will make your blood sugar skyrocket. I've got no doubt that part of the reason America has such a health crisis right now is our obsession with starches!

I'm sure by now you've figured out that your keto diet will consist primarily of meat, cheese, nuts, and any products coming thereof. However, there's a bit of a devil in the details here. First off, be sure that you're eating more than a fair amount of leafy greens. These are your primary source of vitamins and important nutrients, and make a great vehicle for a variance. Meat and cheese can get repetitive. Vegetables, however, can be prepared in any number of different ways!

Also, it can be tempting to cut corners and eat ketogenically solely on beef franks and Vienna sausage. However, avoid processed foods. They are absolutely loaded to the brim with sodium and all sorts of other disgusting things which can make your blood sugar skyrocket. By eating fresh meats and cheeses, you can ensure that you aren't ingesting way too much sodium. You're also making your time on Keto far more enjoyable- we all know fresher food tastes better, and on keto, it costs about the same. So embrace it! Eat fresh deli meats whenever possible.

One last thing: fried food is generally not okay because it's almost always fried in breadcrumbs or a wheat-based batter. This, obviously, can add unnecessary carbs to your diet.

Some people, when they do keto, try to mimic their current eating style by finding replacement foods for their usual foods. This may or may not be the thing you want to do. It's possible, for example, that by making a delicious keto pizza, you get cravings for real pizza, and likewise for any keto sweet replacements. However, there's also the possibility that these can make your transition easier. I'm not going to label these as a do eat or do not eat. It depends on your personal fortitude and, much like strict keto versus lazy keto, what you're trying to do for yourself. If you want keto to be a holistic lifestyle change for the long-term, it may be worth looking. If you just want to hit a goal weight, it may be best to avoid these, as it will take your eyes off of the prize.

Those are basic rules for eating even on while keto. They can keep you happy and healthy as you try to chug your way through your weight loss.

CHAPTER 8

Tips for Eating Out on Keto

One of the hardest things about starting a new diet can be learning to eat in public while you're on it. This process can be painstaking but it doesn't have to be. There are some things that you'll kind of grow into as you learn how keto works and figure out intuitively what you're going to be able to eat - and likewise, what you won't be able to eat.

However, here are some general tips for different cuisines that I've discovered.

American food is a breeze, fortunately. If you go to a steakhouse, you can order any given meat on the menu. Steamed broccoli is always a safe side, and you can salt or butter it to your content. If they don't have any other keto friendly sides, just double up on steamed broccoli.

Diners are easy as well. Often, diners are willing to replace hash browns and other foods that aren't particularly keto friendly with a different side. The classic breakfast of eggs and bacon or sausage is a great go-to, and nothing beats a good steak and eggs.

Coffeehouses are increasingly becoming prevalent as a part of the daily grind. Unfortunately, dropping everything that you know and love - like your caramel macchiato - can be a massive pain. However, you don't have to give it up entirely, fortunately! You can easily get a coffee with cream and sugar-free vanilla syrup. If you want your espresso fix, then espresso is perfectly keto. You can get a Caffè Americano with cream and sugar-free vanilla and it will taste a fair bit like the milky coffee drinks you know and love while clocking in at very few calories.

Mexican food can be harder to eat on Keto. It can be really tempting to eat chips and salsa but you need to resist that temptation and tough through the meal! Your waistline will thank you later. One thing you can always get at a Mexican restaurant is a taco salad. Simply ask that they hold the shell and you'll be all set.

Vietnamese food can be really hard to eat on Keto. Your best option if you're going out to eat Vietnamese is simply to get pho without any noodles.

Japanese food is absolutely delicious, centered around freshness and delicate flavors. However, eating Japanese food while maintaining your keto status can be a difficult task in and of itself. The best option is almost always going to be sashimi. Sashimi is simply super fresh raw fish, and super delicious, too. You'll hardly have something better in your life, so it's well worth ordering in lieu of sushi.

Chinese food is almost impossible to eat out on, unfortunately. Avoid going to

Chinese restaurants as much as you can. If you must, then avoid anything with a sauce as the sauces often contain cornstarch. Cornstarch is loaded with carbs. They also frequently contain sugar.

Italian food is likewise ridiculously hard - the core of Italian dining lies in pasta and bread products. Needless to say, it's almost impossible to find keto food to eat when you're at an Italian restaurant. If you're forced to eat at an Italian restaurant, do what you can to find something based around meat and cheese with minimal sugars and starches.

It's impossible to cover every cuisine, but these are the ones I have the most experience with. I hope that these tips aid you with eating out!

Conclusion

Thank for making it through to the end of this book, let's hope it was informative and able to provide you with all of the tools you need to achieve your goals whatever they may be.

The next step is to take all of this and apply it to your personal life. Conquer keto and conquer your figure!

Finally, if you found this book useful in any way, a review on Amazon is always appreciated!

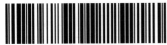

Made in the USA
Lexington, KY
29 December 2017